# CBD

## FOR WOMEN

by Rebecca Valentine

# Contents

**Conclusion** ..................................................................................**79**

# Introduction

In the past 5 years, the market has exploded with interest about cannabinoids. Specifically, the cannabinoid CBD is being raised as a possible remedy for everything from joint pain to depression. Cannabinoids are a very hot topic, and people are asking if they help with certain ailments. In this book I attempt to explain the truth about CBD and the conditions it treats, to the best of my knowledge and the published research today. I firmly believe that CBD is not just another herbal supplement. It is an alternative medication that can help all parts of the body.

As it pertains to females, CBD is being viewed as a promising and intriguing potential health supplement and remedy for a number of health concerns. Women deal with a set of health and fitness considerations that are unique from men. We have a different hormonal structure which manifests both during reproductive years as well as in menopause. We are more prone to inflammation caused by things like arthritis, and to autoimmune diseases like multiple sclerosis. We are more than twice as likely to be diagnosed with depression than men. The list goes on and on.

When we look at all of the systems in our bodies, it is when they are balanced that we are healthiest. Everything in our body is a balance, with many opposites and forming homeostasis. Everything has to be balanced, or in homeostasis, to remain well. It is when balance is lost that a long and unpredictable domino-effect of health issues begins.

The mix of hormones in womens bodies work through a system known as "dynamic balance" - if something is changed in the body, everything will be shifted. Call it the butterfly effect of health. It is not possible to move one part of the body without another part being affected.  The body then has to find its homeostasis again. When there is a shifting in the body, the body becomes ill.

If you are unhealthy, you may choose to visit your doctor, who is likely to prescribe medication. The medication is typically designed to deal with the symptoms. However, the prescribed medication we get from our doctor treats only one condition, not all the symptoms that the condition is causing. Nor does it always treat the underlying condition. The prescribed medication can cause side effects that make you visit the doctor again and you are given another medication to treat that. You might go



Rebecca Valentine

back to treat another condition and suddenly you are weighted down with medication. The system of the body is under so much stress that something breaks.

Pharmaceutical drugs typically work at the level of the symptoms, not often the systems which cause enormous strain on your physiology. CBD, on the other hand, is a naturally-occuring, plant-based compound. CBD may have the potential to address the whole body in a new way and make it healthy again. It works in a holistic way treating the whole body, and the systems that operate within it, rather than separate issues or symptoms.

CBD is transforming the world of holistic therapies, especially where women are concerned. The simple truth is that cannabinoids have the capacity to relieve many illnesses, or at least provide effective therapy for conditions women live with. They can vastly improve women's health and ease some of the unpleasant issues that are individual to each woman. Conditions like premenstrual tension, hormonal imbalances and period cramps. This book will address specific conditions explaining what they are and how cannabinoids can help improve the symptoms of these conditions. Why is CBD such a popular choice of alternative medication? Read on to find out more.

**Author's note:** Always seek the opinion of a medical professional if you are attempting to treat medical conditions, or need to understand the interaction between CBD and medical or health concerns or other drugs you are taking. The information shared in this book should not be considered a substitute for the advice of a qualified medical professional.

# CBD for Anxiety

CBD is a natural compound that helps to reduce anxiety. Anxiety is a condition that makes a person feel shaky and suffer with nerves. Going out of the house may even be feared by sufferers. Stress and anxiety can be brought on by different things. It may cause sweaty hands, clammy forehead, fast pulse, shallow breathing and other symptoms. Panic attacks are common in anxiety sufferers and the person may feel as though they are dying, even though they are not. CBD oil reduces anxiety in women. It makes them relax, thus taking the edge off stress and helping the overall system inside the body.

Extracted from the cannabis plant, CBD oil binds to receptors in the brain, easing the symptoms of anxiety. Women find that they are able to do the things they couldn't before. Walking into a crowded room doesn't seem as frightening. Things that brought about stress now seem easier to cope with thanks to CBD oil.

Numerous research has discovered that CBD relieves anxiety in people who have not been diagnosed with a mental illness. Studies show that it relieves anxiety that was induced in a research based experiment of sufferers with social phobia, reports Loflin et al. (2017)

## Social Phobia

Social phobia is brought about when an anxiety sufferer leaves the home or goes into an environment where communication is required. For serious social phobia sufferers, they may have difficulty going to work because it means they have to mix with other people.

Talking and communicating to others in a group situation can bring about anxiety, even for those who manage stress and anxiety well. The fear of actually leaving the home to go out into a social environment can bring about huge panic. Some people isolate themselves and keep themselves locked inside their homes for fear of mixing with others. CBD can bring that level of anxiety down, helping people achieve things or thrive in settings they could not before.

# Large Numbers Of Anxiety Sufferers

A large proportion of the American population suffers from anxiety, making it the most well-known mental illness in the U.S. Women are more than twice as likely to experience clinical-level anxiety than men, and their anxiety can usually begin at an earlier age. Anxiety is also connected with other mental health problems such as depressed mood and insomnia. It is made worse by caffeine and alcohol use. Since CBD is completely natural, it provides a good form of therapy rather than caffeine, alcohol or other dangerous and potentially addictive substances.

# Five main kinds of anxiety disorder

There are five main kinds of anxiety disorder including:

## Generalized Anxiety Disorder

Generalized Anxiety Disorder is often abbreviated to GAD. This condition brings with it excessive worry that carries on for no apparent reason, especially to everyday events. Individuals with the condition worry about finances, family life, employment or education. They may find using CBD eases their symptoms and stops excessive worrying. Since excessive worrying is part of this condition CBD may take the edge off anxiety and stop the intrusive thoughts.

## Obsessive Compulsive Disorder

Obsessive Compulsive Disorder is characterized by unwanted or intrusive thoughts that the person acts out as a repetitive behavior. CBD may help to ease a person's mind when they feel compelled to carry out obsessions. It may prevent a person from carrying out obsessions. Furthermore, it can stop the intrusive thoughts that occur before the obsession has been carried out.

## Social Anxiety Disorder

Social Anxiety Disorder is a condition that causes embarrassment and fear of scrutiny in public places. It may cause the sufferer to avoid public situations. Therefore, taking CBD may help a sufferer face public situations and reduce the anxiety associated with this. CBD might help the person feel calm enough to talk when faced with public situations and events.

## Post Traumatic Stress Disorder

Post Traumatic Stress Disorder is a condition that occurs due to a past traumatic event. It is often seen in victims of war or soldiers. It affects sleep, causes nightmares or reliving a specific event. CBD may help with flashbacks and reduce the panic associated with them. It may reduce anxiety felt with past events.

## Panic Disorder

Panic Disorder is a condition that is characterized by intense feelings of panic and panic attack. The sufferer worries that they will have another panic attack which can make them even more anxious. Panic attacks might be helped with CBD in reducing the symptoms experienced. CBD may help a sufferer to breathe more easily and avoid going into panic mode.

## Racing Thoughts

Suffering from anxiety is a continuous struggle of overwhelming negative thoughts. Each thought feeds the other thought and soon the mind starts racing. In this mode, it is hard to stop the spiral of racing thoughts and to bring the sufferer back to the present moment. However, CBD helps women to calm down and relax, thus taking the edge off their worries. Cannabinoids may help women relax so much that their mind naturally stops running away with them and their thoughts become more positive. The relaxation experienced may be enough to stop the mind from racing.

# Be Sure You are Using THC-Free CBD

Anxiety sufferers need to know exactly what they are getting in their cannabinoid, because the last thing you want is a mood-altering drug if that is not what you are looking for.

Generally speaking, CBD does not contain THC. With that said, there can be types of CBD that contain traces of THC, and types of CBD that don't, but the industry standard is that a correctly-processed line of CBD does not contain THC. Always check if the CBD you get contains THC, and ensure it has been made by a reputable manufacturer who has a quality production process, because if yours contains THC it can get you high. If you are not looking for a high, then don't buy CBD containing THC.

Furthermore, if you have mental health problems, especially psychosis then it is advisable to stay away from THC which can cause hallucinations in some people.

In fact, part of the allure of CBD is the very fact that you can experience the potential health benefits of cannabinoids without the potential mind-altering effects. Because of that, I'm not sure why people would seek out the THC-heavy versions of CBD.

Depression and anxiety is aggravated by decreased amounts of serotonin, a neurotransmitter that plays a massive effect on mood. SInce CBD can improve serotonin levels it is considered a



Rebecca Valentine

viable choice for treating depression and anxiety. No matter what form it comes in oil, tablets, sweets, mouthspray or other consumables it is a breakthrough in all areas of mental health care.

# Cannabinoids: A Completely Natural Medication

Believe it or not, cannabinoids are produced by your own body. The reason it is believed we get benefit from cannabinoids is because our body is already accustomed to processing it for good purposes, due to the supply of it that it made within the body. The cannabinoids products inside the body are believed to have anti-inflammatory and other positive effects.

Since cannabinoids are completely natural they are a good alternative to conventional medications that come with a range of side effects. In this way they are much safer as they are a natural remedy.

CBD oil is being used, more than ever, for anxiety symptom control. The calming feelings it produces help individuals mental and physical well-being. It is important to note that stress and anxiety are not the same things and alternating CBD oil might be more successful depending on the type of symptoms being dealt with.

Understanding the difference between anxiety and stress will help when seeking a health practitioner for a major condition like anxiety. Thus, cannabinoids can make a huge difference when improving sufferers health and well-being.

The brain chemically produces stress and anxiety as a result of too much specific hormone that increases an individuals feelings of stress and worry. The endocannabinoids system regulates hormones, especially those due to stress - such as adrenaline and cortisol.

## What Is Anxiety? What Is Normal Stress? How Can CBD Help?

We all have stress and anxiety during our life, but it is important to know the difference between an anxiety disorder and anxiety brought about by stress. The sooner that the disorder is recognized, the sooner it can be treated by a professional. Although nothing can replace the advice a professional gives a person, CBD can be used in the interim. CBD can be used for both stress and anxiety. Having said that, if it is a genuine anxiety disorder, it is necessary to seek medical help as soon as possible.

Medical treatments may include a variety of therapies, such as;



Rebecca Valentine

counseling, person-centered, cognitive behavioral, cognitive restructuring and exposure therapies. Some people want relief from their symptoms right away and may choose, with their provider, to take medication known as benzodiazepines. However, as with all medication, benzodiazepines have side effects such as lack of coordination, sleepiness, headaches, feelings of depression and should never be taken with alcohol as the results can be fatal.

The negative side effects of these medications lead people to find alternative treatments for anxiety. For those wanting a more natural treatment, CBD is an answer for a lot of women. However, there is still not a lot known about CBD and more research is needed. Many people are trying cannabinoids on their own terms, but some are worried about the lack of knowledge surrounding it.

People often worry about cannabis products making them high, especially in people who already have problems with their mood. However, CBD alone will not make someone high and it is not psychoactive unless it contains THC, like cannabis. CBD is not like medical marijuana as it only has small trace amounts, if any amount, of THC.

As well as the relaxing properties of CBD, cannabinoid products are taken from industrial hemp plants, rather than marijuana. Hemp plants do not have active levels of THC, but contain more CBD. Due to this, CBD products derived from hemp are legally accepted in the United States and are recognized for their relaxing and calming properties.

People suffering from anxiety disorders or stress may benefit from a frequent, careful, and consistent amount of CBD to remove some of the negative feelings.

Stress is often unpredictable, especially when something unexpected occurs. Therefore, people use CBD oil as the stress arises and choose the fastest delivery method. The quickest way of ingesting CBD is by an Ecig or sublingual CBD oil drops. Ecigs are largely unstudied, however, and we hesitate to recommend anyone begin using them who is not already using ecigs.

People suffering chronic stress on a daily or other regular basis, may find taking CBD frequently more beneficial. CBD oil may help in relieving pain and anxiety.

There is encouraging research that has begun to back up cases about CBD and anxiety. A few investigations demonstrate that CBD decreases constant anxiety with muscle spasms, joint inflammation, and nerve pain according to a recent report in the 'Journal of Experimental Medicine' and 'European Journal of Pain'. The two studies found reduced pain or joint inflammation levels with CBD. Welty clarifies that CBD oil likely improves the impact of pain soothing drugs (like Tylenol or Advil)- However on its own, may not decrease pain.  All things considered, there truly isn't sufficient research yet to know for certain if CBD is successful in any case. There are not enough examinations and case hypotheses and they are not structured well enough. The issue is not with the promising results from such studies, but rather that people are not using a well-tested medication and as such, not much is known about the safety of it.

It is not evident how or why CBD can help with reducing stress, in spite of the fact that the medication has an outstanding calming impact. It is thought to work directly with the endocannabinoid framework in the cerebrum. That end cannabinoid framework, which effects the focal sensory system, impacts neurological experiences like delight, memory, and focus. In any case, we may soon have an authoritative answer. Investigations for pain and discomfort are progressing using new pharma-grade CBD. They will demonstrate to professionals whether the medication is working.

# CBD for Fibromyalgia

Fibromyalgia is a painful disease, and more than twice as likely to strike women than men. It causes joints and the entire body to be sore and painful, causing major quality of life issues for people afflicted by it.

If you are afflicted by fibromyalgia, then I don't need to tell you about the flare-ups that can cause everything from stiffness to joint pain to overwhelming fatigue.

Fibromyalgia also causes musculoskeletal pain, exhaustion and cognitive impairment. There is no cure for this pain condition, and treatment plans look at decreasing pain. Women are often diagnosed in their 30s or early 40s, but it is common for them to have had episodes of some pain much earlier in life.

Due to the lack of clear medical conclusions regarding medical conditions like fibromyalgia, it is highly suggested to seek professional advice before using any alternative form of therapy, including cannabinoids. Having said that, there is some research to suggest that CBD does work for fibromyalgia. Individual testimonies are very positive surrounding pain reduction when using cannabinoids for fibromyalgia, and others swear by CBD's ability to improve stiffness and even fatigue.

In the United States, there is a pain epidemic and fibromyalgia is a large part of that. According to the CDC, more than 20% of adults report chronic pain of some sort. There are no treatments that are 100% beneficial for the majority of fibromyalgia sufferers, and financially there is plenty of incentive to discover a treatment that is best for easing pain and other symptoms. The amount of lost quality time at work and with friends and loved ones is staggering.

There is strong and increasing personal evidence that CBD works for fibromyalgia sufferers. Still, there is a gap between the anecdotes and broad mainstream use, largely because the healthcare community focuses on the tried-and-true treatments that have stood the test of time. Doctors seem interested when people tell them of their success with CBD, but until there is scientific proof it won't be prescribed by most.

Currently there are over 10 million people in the U.S that have Fibromyalgia and although traditional medications are available, many people do not want to take them because of the side effects. According to a survey in 2014, patients claimed that CBD provided much more pain relief than FDA approved medication. I hope such surveys are replicated and expanded, to add validity to CBD as one possible treatment.

Although CBD is not a miracle cure and should never be presented as one, many people with fibromyalgia have found relief from the condition by using CBD. And because fibromyalgia treatment is really about pain management, the prescription alternative often tends to be opioids. As we all know, opioids present a whole host of new problems, so any more natural remedy is absolutely worth trying.

Traditional medications used for fibromyalgia are known for long term severe side effects. The most commonly prescribed medicines for fibromyalgia, like Cimbalta, can be hard on the gut and entire intestinal tract and cause other side effects. We mentioned opioids, which are highly-addictive. Compared to such treatments, CBD oil seems far better for a person's health and well-being. Additionally, CBD is not addictive and is not possible to get addicted to unlike tranquilizer and pain killers. SInce CBD has a different effect on the endocannabinoid system found in humans, each individual reacts in a different way to it.

A high quality dose of CBD may provide relief from fibromyalgia's painful symptoms, while other people may not notice the results as fast. Frequent doses every day seem to be

                                          Rebecca Valentine

necessary for longer term results, and a time of testing doses is needed to find the correct amount for your needs. When considering the amounts needed for fibromyalgia, it's important to consider the way it is consumed, an individual's weight, how severe the symptoms are and a person's metabolism. Also, pay close attention to the dosage recommendations by the manufacturer.

There is lack of research of how much CBD is required for an individual dose. The general advice is to start low and increase the dose until the correct amount is found.

Since CBD works to activate serotonin receptors, it naturally works to decrease pain levels, maintains body temperature and reduces swelling. Such factors may be at play with the difficult symptoms of fibromyalgia and other pain conditions. According to a 2009 study printed by the NIH, CBD can help with neuropathic pain. Two research studies found that CBD was helpful for treating swelling and neuropathic pain resulting from nerve injuries.

Research is ongoing for treatment of fibromyalgia with CBD. Since cannabinoids work to reduce inflammation in the body and people with fibromyalgia have more inflammation than the average person, cannabinoids may help to decrease the pain. Thus, cannabinoids help to improve quality of sleep and insomnia is often reported in fibromyalgia so taking CBD may help improve sleep, thus helping to heal the body.

Medical researchers do not know exactly why CBD decreases the symptoms of fibromyalgia. They also cannot say with certainty why it helps some individuals but, not others. The way CBD works for pain relief is best described in the way it acts in the brain. It disturbs the nerve pathways that send pain messages to the brain and body.

CBD also has an anti-inflammatory action that helps decrease heat and inflammation caused by injury or disease. Thus, reducing pain.

# The Endocannibnoid System

As we begin talking about fibromyalgia and other pain and inflammation conditions, it is important to talk about the endocannabinoid system and CBDs effect on it. Endogenous cannabinoids are made in the body and aid homeostasis of the nervous response system. The ECS reacts to the inner cannabinoids as well as knowing and responding to cannabinoids from outside sources. When CBD goes through the bloodstream, it reactions positively with ECS receptors. This may fight feelings of stress and anxiety, and even pain, through its encounter with the endocannibinoid system.

That brings us to fibromyalgia. While it is a disease that is still being understood, there is a school of thought that suggests it may be cause, at least in part, by a an endocannabinoid deficiency. If your ECB system cannot regulate and balance various chemicals and systems, then the result could easily be pain, inflammation, stiffness, and other things manifested by fibromyalgia. While unproven from a medical study standpoint, there is a valid theory emerging that replenishing the ECB system with CBD could help fibromyalgia and other pain conditions.

# CBD for Smoking Cessation

Womens' relationship to tobacco and smoking is complex. The federal government found that women typically do not get as " hooked" to nicotine as men do, but rather smoke in response to stress, mood, or social cues. Interestingly, though, women have less success when they try to quit smoking. This could be related to any number of things – post-cessation weight gain, mood swings, etc. Females typically experience a relapse rate that is more than 30% higher than men when trying to quit smoking.

Anyone who has ever tried to give up smoking knows how difficult it is. The cravings are extremely difficult to cope with wanting a cigarette, but not being able to have one. Yes, there are nicotine patches, gum, inhalers and other forms of nicotine replacement, but they do not replace a cigarette. It can be extremely difficult coping with the anxiety brought about by giving up smoking, which creates an incredibly strong trigger that drives someone back to cigarettes or e-cigs. Especially in the first few days to weeks, the urges can be all-consuming. However, cannabinoids have once again shown intriguing promise in improving nicotine cravings without the need to actually use nicotine.

Note that using cannabinoids vs. actual cannabis is a huge distinction here. Cannabis has been recognized as an abuser's drug for a long time. However, a number of studies published in the biomedical literature demonstrate that the plant or its compounds have been successful in treating addiction. A more recent review shows the latest evidence on the important role of the endocannabinoid system in controlling addictive behaviors. Animal research has reinforced an important role of the ECB system in psycho and neuro addictive behavior. To study the evidence more deeply, one walks away with at least an interim conclusion that medications which are CB2 receptor agonists - critical to the ECB systems - may help in addictions like cocaine use and nicotine addiction. Observational studies were also carried out and subsequently publish that show a link that cannabis might be a substitute in place of harmful drugs, including alcohol.

According to research published by the World Health Organization which corroborates decades of research gains, tobacco has over 7,000 dangerous chemicals, at minimum 250 of these are harmful for health and at least 69 can cause cancer. There are numerous medical conditions that arise through smoking including the obvious emphysema and lung cancer links, but also breath shortage, asthma, lung infections, coronary heart disease, heart attack, stroke and the list goes on.

A WHO study showed that tobacco is the main preventable reason for death around the world, killing almost 6 million people a year and leading to economic loss estimated to be over half a trillion dollars.

Basically, if you don't smoke, don't start. If you already smoke, try to quit.

In the most recent report from Global Tobacco Surveillance System which collects information from 22 countries accounting for almost 60 percent of global population, researchers found that there were nearly 1,300 million cigarette smokers in those countries. Of those, nearly 205 million had tried to give up smoking in the last year. According to American Cancer Society, only 4-7% of smokers are able to quit in any given attempt without any medical interventions – that is a pretty low success rate. 25% of smokers can quit and remain this way for 6 months or longer with medication.

As noted earlier, women typically experience a higher relapse rate than men when trying to quit smoking.

# Cannabinoids and Addiction?

Cannabinoids work by easing the symptoms of withdrawal and making a person feel more relaxed and calmer. Thus, being able to deal with the effects of withdrawal more easily. No matter what the person is addicted to, cannabinoids could help them overcome the unpleasant symptoms of withdrawal. Furthermore, CBD can help some people remain free of their addiction so they won't relapse as easily.

Some encouraging proof recommends that CBD use may help individuals to stop smoking. A pilot study done for Addictive Behaviors found that inhalers with CBD helped smokers to quit. They smoked fewer cigarettes than expected, and even eliminated their yearnings for nicotine. A similar study which compared the findings, distributed in Neurotherapeutics, concurred. It suggested that CBD could be a promising treatment for individuals with narcotic dependence issue.

The analysts noticed that CBD decreased symptoms related with substance use abuse. These included uneasiness, state of mind related manifestations, agony, and a sleeping disorder. More research is needed in this emerging field of study, yet these discoveries propose that CBD may avoid or decrease withdrawal side effects. Since cannabinoids are completely natural and not addictive, users do not have to worry about becoming addicted to another substance.

# CBD for Alcohol Withdrawal

Continuing on the addiction train-of-thought, there is also promise that CBD can assist with alcoholism treatment in some of the same ways it can assist smoking cessation. Alcoholism and alcohol dependency are hardly gender-specific problems, but they affect women in a unique way. Because of womens' lower tolerance to alcohol for a variety of reasons, they typically experience alcohol problems at an earlier stage than men. Furthermore, the incidence of alcohol problems for females appears to be increasing.

CBD can be very helpful for post-acute withdrawal caused by imbalance in the body due to consuming too much alcohol. It is showing the ability in some to reduce the anxiety and restlessness that is often a part of mild to moderate withdrawal. This alternative medication appears to only help with mild to moderate withdrawal and should not be used for severe withdrawal where a medical professional must be seen.

Given the choice, CBD is much better for alcohol withdrawal than marijuana since it contains no THC. If a person has already been addicted to alcohol or other substances, they don't want to replace that with another potential addiction. Therefore, using marijuana alone is not recommended.

How CBD works with alcohol addiction is similar to how we described it working on nicotine addiction, above. CBD brings balance to the body helping alcohol withdrawal, potentially reducing cravings and creating more stability. CBD is believe by many to have antiaddictive properties and promote recovery from addiction. It also helps those with compulsive behaviors stop those behaviors, in the event that alcohol dependency is closely tied to other habits and triggers.

The inability to regulate GABA, the neurotransmitter that is known to block some brain impulses, is found in people with alcohol withdrawal. Because GABA receptors are overstimulated when someone is using alcohol, an abrupt abstinence from alcohol has the effect of create an imbalance in the GABA receptors.

Similarly, the other primary neurotransmitter that exists along with GABA is glutamate. Alcoholics usually have more glutamate in their systems which makes it hard to relax and people are hypervigilant.

                                    Rebecca Valentine

Where does CBD come in? The NIH found that cannabinoids can have a modulating effect on both GABA and glutamate levels. However, it should be noted that inconsistency was observed in how it might affect different people, so there was no conclusive observation that applied to the entire population.

CBD also reduces inflammation removing a major road block to the production of good chemicals. It repairs activated stress as it is a complete antioxidant. Furthermore, it can reduce the panic people feel when in alcohol withdrawal. It improves the bodies response to stress and has a long term rebalancing effect on the body. CBD helps with withdrawal and prevents from cravings in the future. If the brain chemistry is not properly balanced then it will cause symptoms of cravings.

# CBD for Anemia

Anemia is a health concern that affects hundreds of millions of women all over the world. According to the NIH, women are roughly twice as likely to be afflicted by Anemia than men. In patient forums, the number of anemic women outnumber men by nearly 5:1, suggesting that females may experience more pronounced symptoms. A spike in prevalence occurs in the 30s and 40s, and then again as subjects age past 70.

When the blood has very low red blood cell counts, it leads to Anemia. Therefore, if your red blood cells don't contain enough haemoglobin, you will be at risk of developing anemia. Statistics from the World Health Organization show that around the world, anemia sufferers number 1.62 billion people which is 24.8% of the world's population. The figure is much less in the United States, but the gender prevalence for women holds true.

Standalone anemia is not the only thing that can cause a low red blood cell count – it can also be caused by inflammatory diseases or even certain cancers. The red blood cells are important because they bring oxygen from the lungs to different areas of the body. Hemoglobin is a protein rich in iron that makes the blood red. The condition may be short or long term and mild to severe if not treated correctly.

When hemoglobin is reduced within the body, it is impossible to carry enough oxygen to certain parts of the body. This may lead to stress, insomnia, tiredness and other symptoms. A sufferer might have weakness, fatigue, pale skin, rapid or irregular heartbeat, limited endurance and stamina, difficulty breathing, lack of stability and feeling dizzy, brain fog or difficulty concentrating, not being able to maintain body temperature as in cold feet and hands, headaches and stress.

At first anemia might be mild, but if the symptoms carry on without treatment for months or years, it becomes much more severe.

Anemia does not have one specific reason for its cause. Certain diseases also result in a low red blood cell count. Anemia can result from injuries or conditions like menstruation, peptic ulcers, hemorrhoids, gastritis and cancer as well as others.

There are a lot of ways of treating anemia. Most frequently, the doctor will advise treatment depending on the severity of the anemia. There are some natural forms of treatment for anemia also.

CBD might not treat anemia directly, but it has been shown to be effective in treating pain, fatigue, mood swings, and other symptoms related to anemia. By triggering the serotonin receptors in our bodies, CBD can allow an anemia sufferer to deal with the symptoms and focus on treating the root cause of the disease.

In addition to decreasing the symptoms of anemia, CBD appears to promote a healthy gut too. Cannabinoids contain promising medicinal qualities like anti-inflammatory, anti-anxiety, pain relief, and antipsychotic agents that can bevery helpful in limiting the symptoms of anemia.

# CBD for Multiple Sclerosis

Multiple Sclerosis (MS) is a worldwide condition that affects women at a rate that is 3 to 4 times has high as in men. It tends to be most prevalent in the northern climates. With regard to CBD and MS, the research is still evolving but showing promising results in many patients.

## What is meant by MS (Multiple Sclerosis)

Multiple sclerosis is a condition where the body's framework attacks the focal sensory system (CNS). The precise reason for MS is not exactly understood, yet it might be the consequence of a combination of hereditary and ecological elements. At present, MS influences about 2.3 million individuals in the U.S., most patients are analyzed between the ages of 20-50. It's unknown why the symptoms are more aggressive in some than others. Manifesting MS can range from a slight limp and some numbness to near-total debilitation at times.

Like so many other inflammatory and autoimmune diseases, the symptoms of MS "flare up" from time to time. Such flares are called exacerbations.

In MS, the defensive protection around nerve strands, called myelin, ends up damaged leading to patches of scars. This damage causes the central nervous system to miss brain signals resulting in a wide range of symptoms. As noted before, symptoms vary greatly. A few people experience mild symptoms like fatigue, while others experience pain, involuntary muscle pressure and fits, vision problems, memory loss and in the most severe cases partial or complete loss of movement.

CBD is becoming a topic of much talk in the circles of MS patients. CBD seems to show signs of improving many of the symptoms as it works to repair damage to the central nervous system. People with MS often report improvements in their symptoms after taking a short course of CBD. While it is a promising development for long term for sufferers of Multiple Sclerosis, it definitely should be discussed with the doctor first. Any CBD-based therapy should be done in conjunction with your medical professional's advice and other courses of treatment.

                                    Rebecca Valentine

# CBD for the Different Types of MS

## Relapsing Remitting:

This is the most widely recognized type of MS, around 85 percent of MS patients get a diagnosis of RRMS. Individuals with RRMS experience brief flare-ups or times when their illness is worse, followed by times of abatement where no symptoms are experienced.

During flare ups CBD may be taken intermittently to help with symptoms during this time. However, patients with MS may need to take conventional medication alongside this alternative source and must always discuss with a doctor first.

## Secondary Progressive:

For individuals with this type of MS, symptoms get better after a period of time with or without flare-ups. The vast majority diagnosed with RRMS progress to SPMS.

Very good results have been seen in patients with MS taking CBD. People who have mobility problems, hip and leg pain improve with this alternative medication. When pain is found in the hips, legs and it causes mobility problems, canniboidal can be taken as a suppository. The suppository goes directly into the nervous system around the spine and down into the legs. It seems to work more quickly as a suppository compared with any other form of ingestion, although I do not have hard statistics for that claim.

## Primary Progressive:

This type is quite rare and only occurs in around 10 percent of MS patients. Gradually getting worse from the moment of diagnosis, it has no flare-ups or times of remission.

Cannabinoids can help with spasticity in MS. However, research to date no evidence has been found that it will help disease modifying therapy.

## Progressive Relapsing:

This uncommon type of MS happens in around five percent of patients. Symptoms get worse from onset, with severe regression and no improvement of condition. In this case, CBD is probably less of an option than medical marijuana, for comfort and pain management.

## CBD oil with Multiple Sclerosis:

Dr. Ben Thrower is a doctor at the Shepherd Center in Atlanta, GA, a medical professional with some expertise in research and restoration for individuals with illnesses like multiple sclerosis. As indicated by Dr. Hurler, MS patients find that the full-range CBD medication is the most useful for treating both spasticity and pain. "Many of our MS patients have used hemp-based CBD items with 0.3 percent THC." Thrower said. For helping with spasticity/fits or reducing pain (focal neuropathic pain), I have discovered that most patients need higher THC doses.

Since THC is a well-known pain reliever, that may be why products high in THC are well known for treating MS symptoms. Be that as it may, Thrower said a few patients do discover help with "low-THC, CBD products". With respect to undesirable symptoms, Thrower said there are not many, and they're rare. "CBD/THC items will in general be far less steadying than Baclofen or Tizanidine, which are [muscle relaxants] customarily used for spasticity.

In spite of the fact that there isn't much proof suggesting that CBD or different cannabinoids can heal nerve pain in the long term, research has progressed.

# One Story of CBD oil for MS:

Devin Garlit, who has regressive multiple sclerosis, uses CBD items alongside his recommended MS medicine, Tysabri. The CBD has been especially useful in dealing with his symptoms. "CBD has helped me massively with pain and fits," Garlit said. "I still have side effects, but they are easier to endure than they were before I began using CBD".

In spite of the fact that it required Garlit some investment to see whether the CBD was working, he says that it's been useful. Friends noticed that he looked better and was able to get out of the home easier and accomplish more. That was when Garlit noticed how well CBD was working and started to welcome the impacts of CBD. Garlit uses a full-range CBD tincture, taking around one milliliter orally consistently, and that routine has been significant. A massive turning point was taking CBD regularly. Garlit also said that he has not encountered any negative symptoms from the CBD.

There are no concerns identified with taking CBD for multiple sclerosis. Nonetheless, on the grounds of THC and CBD combined, by all accounts, to be a prevalent and successful

                                   Rebecca Valentine

treatment for MS, a few patients might need to stay away from the psychoactive impacts of high doses of THC. On the off chance that you need to abstain from high levels of THC, it's ideal to begin with CBD that has low THC-to-CBD proportions, for example, most full-range CBD oils.

When considering using CBD for a specific ailment, it is best to do so under the advise of a specialist. This is, even more important in the event that you are taking different prescribed medication. In case CBD does not react well to the medication or causes side effects.

# CBD for Pain Relief:

I wrote earlier about the promise of CBD and fibromyalgia, and the good news is that the same reasons why it may help fibromyalgia may apply to other pain-related condotions.

## Arthritis

We have all heard about people with arthritis, and you may possible have it yourself. Arthritis is a combination of swelling and tenderness in joints, but for the sufferer it simply means that your joints are painful and stiff. Arthritis most commonly affects us as we age, but certain types of it can affect the young as well.

Generally speaking, joint inflammation has been cited as the main reason why people are unemployed in the United States, affecting more than 50 million Americans. There are two predominant types of joint pain.

Rheumatoid joint inflammation (RA) is actually immune

 

system illness where an individual's body assaults their joints, causing aggravation and soreness. RA normally affects the hands and feet and causes difficult, swollen, and hardened joints.

Osteoarthritis (OA) is a degenerative illness that affects joint ligaments and bones, causing pain and inflammation. It regularly affects the hip, knee, and thumb joints.

Animal testing suggests that CBD could treat joint pain and alleviate the related inflammation pain. A recent report found that CBD diminished pain and swelling in rodents by influencing the manner in which the brain receptors react to improvements.

A recent report found that a cannabis-based mouth spray called Sativex alleviated joint inflammation.   While discoveries so far have been empowering, more research is needed to affirm that CBD oil is a successful treatment for joint inflammation. Ultimately, I think the proof will emerge, but for now I have to appropriately caveat that advanced medical testing has been limited.

# Chronic Pain:

Many people around the world live with the more general chronic pain. Aside from fibromyalgia and arthritis, there are many who simply are living with pain. It appears that CBD may help some sufferers deal with the pain.

Cannabinoids join themselves to particular receptors in an individual's brain and body, including an all-important CB2 receptor. The CB2 receptor plays an important role of overseeing pain and inflammation. It is unclear whether cannabinoids actually join the CB2 receptors and bolster them, or encourage the body to produce more and stronger CB2 receptors themselves. Either way, some scientists believe there is enough from early studies that merits a more in-depth analysis.

Researchers think that, in part, because CBD has an indirect ability to positively impact CB2 receptors, there is promise for CBD and pain. Given the CB2 receptors' moderating ability on pain, anything that can be done to bolster them and the entire ECB system shows promise.

# CBD for Psoriasis

Psoriasis is a condition that affects people all over the world. While it is generally not viewed as a notable women's condition, it is something that enough females suffer from so I decided to write about it.

Women are fortunate to not be as afflicted by psoriasis as men, and when they get it, it generally is not as severe as in men. Still, if you are a female with psoriasis, it is a big deal to you, and CBD could potentially help.

In 2017, the Journal of the American Academy of Dermatology noted that limited studies found promise in the role of cannabinoids in improving the symptoms caused by psoriasis.

As with so many things related to CBD, the small sample size limits the number of valid statistical studies can tell us for sure if it works or not. What we know is that Psoriasis is a very difficult condition to treat, and many of the medicines used to treat it are steroid-based. Enbrel, Remicade, Humira, and Stelara are some of the more common ones. In addition to being steroid-based, they are expensive and cost-prohibitive for anyone who has to foot their own drug bill. Any type of corticosteroid should not be used for long periods of time, and could become less effective as the drug is used more and more.

It stands to reason that psoriasis can be treated by CBD, given that CBD is both an anti-inflammatory and an immune system aide. I see great promise in the link between CBD and psoriasis treatment, but as of today it is mainly anecdotal.

## How to use CBD oil for Psoriasis:

CBD is accessible as an oil or powder, which can be used to make creams or gels that individuals can apply to the skin in the areas affected by joint inflammation. Individuals can likewise take CBD as a tablet, sweet, lollipop or as an oral mouthwash.

# CBD for Female Aging

One could argue that everything I write about is related to female aging! After all, as we get older, we all become more prone to various diseases and conditions. But the general category of age-related health issues warrants a section in my book.

CBD, being a phytocannabinoid and a compound made by the cannabis plant, could be relatively natural way to address many possible aging issues.

As women age in the postmenopausal stage, the prevalence of osteoporosis increases. The battle to keep your bone mass and density is real, and something that all females should be focused on . After the age of 50, bone density decreases dramatically, especially in white females.

You can make sure you are getting enough calcium and exercise to aide your retention of bone density, but there is also a role for cannabinoids. Findings suggest that the activation of

CBD <u>may</u> increase bone density and slow bone loss. The research is new on this but, CBD has been shown to help with osteoporosis.

If CBD helped with bone density alone, it would be a major finding, but there may be other age-related conditions that women can consider it for. Older women suffer from specific problems, they may have joint issues, bladder problems, sciatica, skin conditions and more. However, cannabinoids work on the system we have inside our body that is receptive to cannabinoids.

Older women suffering from hormonal imbalances such as painful periods, thyroids, endometriosis, decreased libido, skin problems and breast tenderness may find CBD helpful. This medication can balance hormones bringing relief from women's pain.

CBD helps to balance the endocrine system which activates different receptors in the brain and body. The activity in the endocrine glands are very receptive to CBD.

With emerging promise for the impact of cannabinoids on so many age-related female health conditions, it is worth watching new studies emerge that can further our understanding of CBD and women's aging.

# CBD for Cancer Treatment

Some people use CBD as part of broader cancer therapy, typically to help deal with the side effects of aggressive cancer treatment. Given the prevalence of cancer nowadays, and the intense battle so many people wage against it, we hope that CBD can emerge as an important tool in the toolset against cancer.

Women experience certain cancers at a rate far greater than men. The most obvious example is breast cancer, which accounts for nearly 25% of all new cancer diagnoses in women. Other common female cancers include colorectal, lung, and skin cancers.

Always talk to your doctors about your cancer treatment before incorporating CBD or any other self-prescribed therapy into your treatment plan. It is way too soon to make any cases for CBD within a cancer treatment regimen, but this is some belief that this compound may help oversee side effects that happen because of cancer or due to treatment.

Likewise, because of the severity of a cancer diagnosis, it is important to work with your team of health professionals to understand all of the possible treatment options. CBD may play a role in that (perhaps to offset side-effects of more proven treatments).

We hear lots of associated between actual medical marijuana and cancer treatment, many to reduce the effects of pain. It is important to not that medical marijuana is not CBD. Unless CBD has THC in it, which is not usually the case, it won't get the user high. When they talk about medical marijuana and pain management in cancer patients, they often are referring to the effects of THC. THC should not be found in properly-processed CBD.

When it comes to the impact on malignant cancer cells, I am not going to make any claims in this book. There is just not enough known about CBD at the moment to say for definite if it effectively treats cancer. Since cancer is such a serious illness, it is best not to grasp for any one "magic" medicine, including CBD or anything else for that matter.

The theory (and it is just a theory right now) on CBD may work on cancer has to do with receptors. There are two types of CBD receptors in our bodies - CB1 receptors (mainly in the brain, but also heart, liver and pancreas) and the CB2 receptors. The CB2



Rebecca Valentine

receptors are closely linked to many systems associated with cancer, control pain, and may play a role in telling cells when to die. Using forms of CBD, a research team lead by Professor Marco Felasca was able to eradicate almost 100% of the cancer in test tubes, but they had low expectations when they moved on to tumors in mice. To their surprise they found that almost 25 to 30 % of mice completely rejected the tumor and were cured. In the remaining mice there was a significant decrease in the size of tumor.

# CBD oil as complementary cancer therapy:

## Appetite Simulation:

Many individuals who are going through disease treatment experience nausea and loss of appetite. These side effects can make it hard for them to maintain a good weight and energy level, important factors in fighting any disease. There is a link to cannabis and the ability to drive appetite, although studies specific to CBD are still evolving.

## Relieving the Pain:

Cancer and its treatment can cause pain. Since CBD works on the

CB2 receptors, which are central to the body's pain signals, CBD may help with pain relief caused by discomfort and inflammation. THC follows up on the CB1 receptors as well, which prove useful for pain arising due to nerve damage.

## CBD take away in cancer treatment:

While CBD is showing promise in the fight against cancer, and especially dealing with the treatment of it, it is important not to overstate the research-to-date. CBD might be a helpful compound for some malignant growth manifestations, but it is very, very early in the medical community's understanding of it.

There is no magic bullet when it comes to cancer. Please do not self-prescribe CBD or any other homeopathic treatment. The stakes are too high.

Cancer treatment should be coordinated by your medical professional, but you can always ask about including alternative therapies.

Women should talk with a specialist before using any type of non-traditional treatment in their fight against cancer.

# CBD for Migraines

Did you know that 80% of migraine sufferers are women? Migraines can have a major impact on our ability to work, parent, and enjoy life in general. Anything we can do to minimize the effects would be a welcomed improvement.

Some women using CBD report that it reduces the indications of certain sorts of cerebral pain. It is only anecdotal at this time. There is little medical proof – through scientific studies --  that CBD oil is viable as a treatment for headaches. All things considered, for individuals who still can't seem to locate a powerful headache treatment, it might be worth considering.

Always buy CBD from a trustworthy source, to guarantee its safety. The legalities of cannabis items, including CBD oil, are evolving rapidly. Individuals may require a prescription to use CBD oil legitimately in their state, depending on where you live and the latest regulatory advances. A specialist can give an individual information on whether it is legal to use CBD oil in their general vicinity.

## Why we might use CBD oil in Migraine treatment

Individuals actually used cannabis for several years to treat headaches and migraines before it became illegal. While there is currently an absence of logical proof about its effectiveness, anecdotal evidence is building. Analysits have proposed that at least one substance present in cannabis may have helpful advantage for cerebral pains, including headaches.

As I have written about with other conditions in the book, there is emerging evidence that CBD oil can diminish irritation and joint pain. By focusing on the same receptors, it might work also with headaches. As the studies come in looking at the viability and reactions of CBD oil, I think that migraines will be an area of likely interest among patients and the medical community.

## CBD Take Away in Migraine Treatment:

As with the other conditions written about in this book, anyone with a serious migraine issue should speak with their physician before trying to self-administer a remedy. Because the typical migraine sufferer is probably on other medications, making sure that all of the treatments fit will together is key.

# CBD for Inflammation Treatment:

Inflammation and many other conditions I have written about go hand-in-hand. In fact, many conditions in our body are simply the presence of inflammation in a place where it should not be. You could make the case that most diseases are, at least in part, inflammation.

Inflammation can be serious. When we consider inflammation, we normally think of conditions like arthritis, joint pain and other joint conditions, but inflammation is also one of the forerunners to coronary illness.

One of the main reasons that we hear so much about inflammation is because of how we eat. The standard American eating regimen (substantial on sugar and grains). Fried foods and other fatty foods cause inflammation, and likewise eating cleaner can help reduce inflammation.

Research into the calming and anti-inflammatory effects of

CBD oil is becoming more widely accepted and looks promising for individuals who experience the ill effects of asthma, multiple sclerosis, Hashimoto's illness, lupus, and even celiac sickness.

Studies have shown that CBD can help reduce inflammation, which could have a far-ranging effect on a number of conditions and maladies that women (and men too) experience in their lifetime.

# CBD for Cardiovascular Treatment:

Coronary illness is one of the main causes of death in the US. While some think of coronary illness as a men's health issue, the number of women who are developing coronary disease is increasing at a disturbing rate. It is especially prevalent in women aged 60 and over.

While a sound eating routine and regular exercise are the best places to begin when fighting coronary illness, CBD oil has appeared to impact some of the reasons for coronary illness. Evidence hints that it lessens blockage in conduits, brings down cholesterol, diminishes the pressure reaction in heart assaults, and decreases circulatory strain. It is unknown if these are direct or indirect effects of CBD, but evidence is mounting.

The NIH found that CBD can have a vasorelaxation effect (it helps your cardiovascular system relax) and can protect against vascular damage caused by external factors. This promising research might be among the most exciting of all research being done on CBD, and we are grateful that organizations like the NIH are investing in it.

# CBD for Epilepsy

Epilepsy is often seen as a predominantly women's health issue. The fact is that men and women get epilepsy at about the same rate – it is just that women are far more likely to have the severity that causes seizures, making it a more visible condition in females.

In the wake of looking into the security and viability of CBD oil for treating epilepsy, the FDA endorsed the utilization of CBD (Epidiolex) as a treatment for two uncommon conditions portrayed by epileptic seizures in 2018. I cannot overstate the importance of this breakthrough, to have an organization as cautious as the FDA endorsing a drug whose active ingredient is CBD.

In the U.S., a specialist can also recommend Epidiolex to treat Lennox-Gastaut disorder (LGS), a condition that shows up between the ages of 3 and 5 years and includes various types of seizures.   They can also prescribe it for Dravet disorder (DS), an



Rebecca Valentine

uncommon hereditary condition that shows up in the first year of life and includes fever-related seizures.

The kinds of seizures that portray LGS or DS have proven hard to control with different sorts of prescriptions. It is important to note that the FDA indicated that specialists couldn't recommend Epidiolex for very young children. A doctor or drug specialist will need to decide the correct measurement dependent on body weight.

# CBD for Bipolar disorder

Women's bipolar disorder behaves different than in men. They tend to be more affected by seasonal fluctuations. They often get it later in life. And they are more prone to the Type II disorder which is begins with extended depressive episodes.

The literature that was reviewed by Loflin et al. 2017 attempted to find a link between CBD and bipolar treatment. When mice were studied who had been given CBD, they were shown to act similarly to those who had been given an antidepressant drug.

Additionally, there are studies being coordinated by the NIH to understand the effects of both medical marijuana and CBD on bipolar disorder. The studies are designed to validated (or not) if the anecdotes that CBD helps with bouts of mania and depression are scientifically-supported.

It is important to note that the number of studies showing a link between CBD and depression treatment is limited. We hope more will be published soon, because the anecdotes suggest that it may help some people.

# CBD for Pre Menstrual Syndrome (PMS)

You are in the middle of a chaotic day when your period comes knocking at the door. You can see the signs a mile away; swelling, acne, cramping, mood swings, anxiety and even constipation. Most women can relate to the changes that periods cause, but more women are turning to CBD to solve those issues.

PMS can happen before or during the time of your period, and it may include breast soreness, cramping, mood swings, anxiety, stomach bloating, severe fatigue, constipation, cravings and basically is no fun whatsoever. Some women experience moderate PMS, but for others it can be quite severe (your genetics influence how bad yours will be). On the horizon though is good news. CBD appears to possible help by interacting with hormones and restoring the natural balance within the body.

Studies are in process, and we hope there will be many useful



Rebecca Valentine

ones published in the near-future.  For now, though, a few things are becoming clearer from the anecdotes.

For some women, CBD is a game-changer by reducing the anxiety associated with PMS. It can help women sleep and relax, and reduce irritation.

For other women, CBD has the even-more physical effect of reducing cramps. Anytime you can reduce cramps with PMS with a natural supplement, you reduce the need for taking harsh aspirin or ibruprofen, a win-win.

# CBD Reference and Background Information

## How do you take CBD?

One of the most basic questions I get is how you take CBD. There are a few common ways.

**Just Swallow it**. You can take the oil the same way you might take cough syrup or liquid Tylenol. It doesn't taste too bad, and this is probably the easiest way to just get it over with. Take it in the morning, after you have had some small breakfast, just in case it might irritate your stomach.

**Mixing with beverages**. Tea is a favorite. Many people like to put their drops of CBD oil into black, herbal, or green tea.  Same goes for coffee..... "Would you like some cream with that? Yes, and sugar, and some CBD."

**Taking in capsulate**. Taking a capsulate form of CBD is just like taking your daily multivitamin, in pill form. Just make sure that the other stuff in the capsule is harmless. The "filler" is usually benign, but worth a read on the ingredients.

**Inhaling in or vaping**. I have to put this on the list for completeness, however there are explicit perils to the lungs and revealed dangers of harmfulness. I want to be clear – I **don't** recommend this way.

**As a topical application** for the skin. This is as simple as applying an ointment or oil to the skin, just like you would with Neosporin or other topicals.

The best plan, if you are a new user, is to begin with an exceptionally low portion and check whether it helps. To be safe, don't use CBD for the first time when you are about to drive or perform dangerous activities.

# Is CBD (Cannabidiol) oil legal or not

Disclaimer: I am not a legal expert, and the rules by country and by state are different. Do your research.

There is a lot of confusion over the legality of CBD oil in some countries. CBD oil is legal in a number of countries, whereas others it is not. In other countries, it might be legal in one district or state, but not in another.

CBD can be extracted from Hemp which has more CBD in, and depending on where it is bought will not have THC in. CBD oils, that have been prepared from the hemp plant, are legitimate to have under the new government law as long as they, contain close to 0.3 percent THC. If CBD is separated from cannabis and contains no THC it is now legal in all states of America. It is when CBD is combined with THC that it becomes illegal. Cannabinoids as a supplement are legal.

CBD with THC in it is believed to be lawful in every one of the states where recreational marijuana use is legal-eight states, including places like California and Colorado. The equivalent goes for states where therapeutic use is permitted; however, from that point, the legitimacy's of CBD gets a little murky.

Laws are always changing, do your own research based on where you plan to buy and use CBD.


# CBD oil does not have the ability to make women high

We should be clear CBD oil won't get women high, the compound in marijuana that causes the trademark psychoactive 'high' is found in THC, not CBD.

Assuming your CBD has been processed correctly, it does not

                                           Rebecca Valentine

get you high.

It is important to caveat, though, that incorrectly-processed CBD could accidentally have some CBD... that is why you need to buy it from a reputable manufacturer. Many of these CBD products are new to the market though and not regulated so it is difficult to know what ingredients they contain.


## How much does a woman usually take?

While the right amount of CBD fluctuates by person and condition, most CBD oil comes in 10 to 15-milligram dosages per one milliliter of oil (the size of a standard dropper). Be that as it may, the genuine measure of CBD can fluctuate massively. The FDA for the most part considers the oil a dietary enhancement-which they don't screen or manage.

"There's no genuine control, and there's no prerequisite for substance or portion in the most part, accessible dispensaries sold or appropriated in the states where it's lawful". Says Timothy Welty, PharmD, chair of the department of clinical sciences at Drake University's College of Pharmacy and Health Sciences.

At first it is best to take 5 or 10 mg of CBD a day for 10 days and after, if it doesn't feel like it is working properly, it is possible to double it to 20mg. Some people find that they develop dry mouth, nausea, drowsiness and headaches as a side effect from CBD.

CBD has a really good overall safety profile unlike other drugs there are no major side effects. The side effects reported include drowsiness, stomach discomfort, sedation, appetite disruption, but these were caused in case studies where people were given very high doses of CBD. Depending on the reason for using CBD, many have found side effects helpful. For example, if you are having problems sleeping, the drowsiness might help.

If you are experiencing side effects it could be because of other prescription drugs you are taking. Therefore, consult with your doctor when using CBD.

## Side Effects of CBD oil:

Small scale studies have discovered that individuals for the most part endure CBD well, yet a few people may encounter mild side effects. These include:

- Tiredness

- Bad Mood

- Queasiness

Clinical preliminaries of Epidiolex, the brand name of the CBD prescription that the United States Food and Drug Administration (FDA) have endorsed to treat epilepsy, did not display any signs of physical dependency.

CBD is legitimate in certain states in the U.S. but, not every one. Individuals should check the laws in their area before buying or taking CBD oil.

A few people may have a hypersensitive response to topical CBD oil, so it is a good idea to apply the oil to a little part of the skin first.

Most people decide to try out cannibanoids first before committing to them long term. As I mentioned before, it is best to try at a time when you are not about to drive or operate any dangerous maneuvers, like working with machinery.

Some might do a short course of CBD, try it for 30 days and build it up in their body. If there is reduced pain, mood stabilization and improvement in sleep then it can be reduced

## Hemp And Cannabis Are Different

Hemp and cannabis may come from the same family, but they are completely different. CBD comes from hemp plants. Hemp can be found in many industries and was even used for rope. It was given as a beverage in the Victorian era to help calm people down. In the 1800's it was a regular part of the pharmaceutical industry. Cannabinoids can be found in the human body and even in breast milk. Farmers would use hemp to help plants and crops grow, but when it was banned in the 1800's they had to stop using it. Grass was rich with hemp and cows would eat it, filling their bodies with the nutritious supplement. Humans would then eat the cows, consuming vital elements needed from hemp. Due to the ban on hemp use in farming, humans are now deficient in hemp which is leading to many medical problems. This deficiency has led to scientists naming  a condition after it called, "Clinical Endocannabinoid Deficiency". The way of treating this condition is to consume CBD supplements. Products rich in hemp may help this condition.

Hemp helps to keep our body balanced and healthy.


## Is CBD Safe To Use While Pregnant?

This is an area where I most definitely say that you should consult your doctor.

When it comes to actual Marijuana, the answer is clearer. Don't use it while pregnant. Marijuana use in women is increasing. There is not enough evidence to say it is safe to use while pregnant. There is some evidence to say marijuana does not allow the babies brain to develop properly.

However, CBD has also **not yet** been shown to be safe during pregnancy or breast feeding. THC crosses over to the breast milk. Since it is not regulated it's important to be careful where you buy it. There is no way of checking how much THC it has in it. Err on the side of caution if using it during pregnancy. It is not safe during pregnancy or breast feeding.

# Female Influencers Of CBD Use

There are numerous female celebrities and well-known endorsers of CBD. People like Kristen Bell have come forward and spoken of their experiences with cannabinoids.

The famous actress takes CBD every day and really believes in the healing properties of the plant. Kristen Bell has said that she takes it every day because of the fact that there are no psychoactive properties so she can enjoy time with her children. Bell is a mother to two children with her husband Dax Shepard and has praised CBD as helping her to cope with the acting industry and stress she experiences.

Chelsea Leyland is working towards cannabis being legalized and suffers from a specific kind of epilepsy known as "Juvenile Myoclonic Epilepsy" since being a teenager. In 2016 Leyland came off her usual prescription anti-seizure medication to use medical cannabis only. Now she is an advocate for medical cannabis.

Jessie Glll, is an RN cannabis nurse who suffered a back injury that led to her setting up a website, MarjuanaMommy.com, where she fights the stigma surrounding marijuana use. She prefers using CBD Living suppositories and finds them helpful for endometriosis pains.

Kimberly Dillon is a chief marketing officer for California's top cannabis brand, Papa & Barkley leading the wellness space. Dillon is also the founder of plantandprosper.co. Dillon is a public speaker on the positive effects of CBD products, including the amount of people who have used it for skin complaints like psoriasis, rashes and dermatitis.

Jessica Catalano is recognized as a top marijuana chef in America. She combines her passion for cooking with her knowledge of cannabis making wonderful medicated dishes. Catalano has benefited many people with health problems. She is known as the "OG Cannabis Chef" for her work in restaurant and bakery.

# Conclusion

There is still a lot not known about CBD but, even so, it is very popular. Although a popular choice of medication, it is not regulated well. By itself CBD won't get you high and it is only when it has large quantities of THC in that it will make a person experience euphoria.

People say CBD can treat everything, but there is not enough data to prove it does treat specific disorders. We don't know what it does to the brain as the long term effects have not been measured. We do not even have specific, factual information on the correct doses to take. CBD products often don't contain what they say on the bottle and might not even contain CBD at all. Even when bottles are tested and shown to contain CBD, the measurement of CBD is very low. The amount needed to treat conditions is much higher than the amount of CBD that is dripped down into the market. Since most people buy CBD from the internet they don't really know what they are getting.

Today coffee shops are even selling drinks with CBD in it. That means you can walk down the street and grab a CBD coffee. When you buy a drink containing cannibinoids you might get a measurement of between 5 to 10 milligrams of CBD, but in reality you would need 30 times that amount to experience the results that researchers have found to be effective in treating anxiety. If you go down the street and purchase a coffee with cannabinoids in, that is still federally illegal in certain states.

Bakeries are experimenting with cannabinoids and in the news a hotel in Essex, UK has just opened dedicated to CBD. People everywhere are talking about the positive benefits cannabinoids are bringing them. If there was ever a time to jump on the bandwagon and try cannabinoids, it is now.

The DEA states that CBD is still federally illegal, but it won't chase after anyone possessing or using it. Because the DEA won't prosecute, anyone from any state can go online or to the store and buy CBD products. The good news is that research is being carried out all the time and hopefully one day it will be regulated and sold only by those who have a license to sell it.

Attitudes towards health care are changing in 2017, the World Health Organization concluded that CBD is not harmful. In January 2018 the World Anti-Doping Agency removed it from its prohibited substances list. In 2018 the Farm Bill legalized CBD and industrial Hemp. We need dispensaries that provide CBD under a regulated fashion. When we understand how to use CBD medicinally we will have much more benefit in the communities.

Finally, note that everything surrounding CBD is changing constantly. It is a very dynamic time for cannabinoids, hemp, CBD, and medical marijuana, as well as other types of alternative therapies. Laws are changing, studies are evolving, proof is emerging on how CBD might interact with all kinds of different conditions. I will do my best to update this book at a regularly frequency, but I advise you to do your own research. In regard to laws, the research should be based on specifically where you live.

And, as I have written so many times in this book that you are probably tired of reading it, always consult your medical professional when attempting to treat your health conditions.

If you have enjoyed this book, I welcome you to leave a review. It would mean a lot to me, and would help future readers too. You can do that here:



Rebecca Valentine